Puberty In Girls : Puberty Questions On Everything Including Sex

Puberty Questions For Girls A Survival Guide

By: Dana Tebow

ISBN-13: 978-1478135661

Publishers Notes

BINDERS PUBLISHING LLC

Disclaimer

This publication is intended to provide helpful and informative material. It is not intended to diagnose, treat, cure, or prevent any health problem or condition, nor is intended to replace the advice of a physician. No action should be taken solely on the contents of this book. Always consult your physician or qualified health-care professional on any matters regarding your health and before adopting any suggestions in this book or drawing inferences from it.

The author and publisher specifically disclaim all responsibility for any liability, loss or risk, personal or otherwise, which is incurred as a consequence, directly or indirectly, from the use or application of any contents of this book.

Any and all product names referenced within this book are the trademarks of their respective owners. None of these owners have sponsored, authorized, endorsed, or approved this book.

Always read all information provided by the manufacturers' product labels before using their products. The author and publisher are not responsible for claims made by manufacturers.

The statements made in this book have not been evaluated by the Food and Drug Administration.

Binders Publishing LLC
7950 NW 53rd Street
Miami,
FL 33166

Dana Tebow

Manufactured in the United States of America

ISBN-13: 978-1478135661

Table of Contents

Dedication

I want to dedicate this book to my daughter who is going through a rough time with puberty. I wrote this book for all the Moms like me helping their teenage daughters understand their body.

CHAPTER 1- PUBERTY; A DEFINITION

Puberty happens naturally; when the body of a child moves into an adult body and becomes ready for reproduction. There are specific signs that will be seen in girl that is entering puberty. These signs are inclusive of growth in her breasts, body odor, hair growth under her arm and on her vagina, acne on her face, as well as the onset of her menstrual cycle.

It is usual for girls to start puberty before boys and some of them even start to show signs of puberty from as early as nine years old. Most girls will start menstruating between the ages of eleven and twelve. Some girls will start showing signs of puberty prior to their eighth birthday and when this happens, it is known as precocious puberty. This is a condition that can be treated and should be definitely be dealt with by a pediatrician.

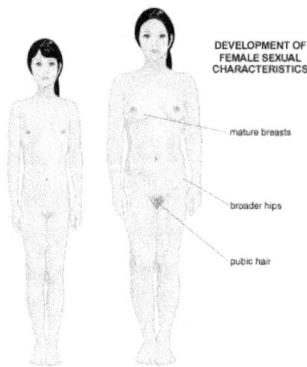

DEVELOPMENT OF
FEMALE SEXUAL
CHARACTERISTICS

mature breasts

broader hips

pubic hair

Those girls who enter puberty either too early or too late are often times very self-conscious about it and may even end up being quite worried and/or depressed and may therefore need some help getting used to the situation. The ones that are slower in getting there should be encouraged and told that it will happen for them soon; when it is the right time for it to happen.

Puberty sometimes come with bursts of anger and moodiness. This is largely due to the hormonal changes that are going on in their bodies that will also impact on their emotions as well as on their bodies. It is very necessary for parents and other caregivers to inform their children about the changes they will be experiencing during this time of their lives, so it will be less scary to them.

CHAPTER 2- YOUR HEIGHT : WHAT HAPPENS TO GIRLS GROWING TALLER

In addition to all the other changes that take place in a girl's body during puberty, growth spurt is also another change that they will experience. By the time a girl gets to the age of nine, she will start gaining approximately seventeen or eighteen percent of her adult height. Their limbs will start growing first, followed by their trunk. When a girl enters puberty, it is usual for her to have the fastest spurt in their growth approximately 6 months prior to them starting their first period.

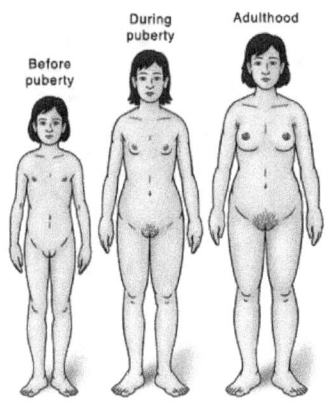

Your height will be checked annually so that the doctor can monitor your growth in order to ensure that you are growing at the rate that you should be growing. The rate of growth in a girl is usually at its highest two years after she has begun puberty. On average, a girl of twelve years old will grow between 4'10 and 5'1, a thirteen year old girl will grow between 5'0 and 5'3. In addition, a fourteen year old girl will grow an average of between 5'1 and 5'4, a fifteen year old will grow between 5'2 and 5'5, while a sixteen year old teenage girl will grow between 5'3 and 5'6, a seventeen year old will to between 5'3 and 5'7 and an eighteen year old can grow to between 5'3 and 5'7 inches tall.

There will be those girls who will get to their adult heights at an earlier age and this, according to psychologists; often times put them at an advantage when they are in junior high school as well as in high school. A part of this is due to the fact that their growth and physical development is said to be very closely related and they therefore have a higher self-esteem than those teenage girls who mature later rather than earlier.

CHAPTER 3- EATING HEALTHY AND MAINTAINING A HEALTHY WEIGHT

Yet another change that a girl will experience during puberty is a change in her weight. Her hips, arms, thighs and buttocks will get bigger. Their eating habits should be carefully monitored, as their nutritional needs will be tied into the changes that are happening in their bodies during this crucial period of their development.

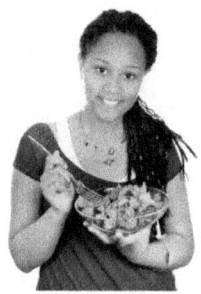

It is very important that their weight be properly maintained so that they will not become obese. To help to maintain the healthy weight of your teenage girl, you should try your best to monitor what they eat when they are around you, as well as to instill proper eating habits in them so that they will make informed food decisions when they are away from you.

To try to ensure that they eat healthily when they are not around you, you can prepare their meals and send it with them to school. This will help with their issue of meal convenience, which is often times what influences a teenager to eat poorly when they are out of the sight of their parents and presented with more bad foods than good foods, such as the foods sold in their school canteen.

In addition, parents and other caregivers should also try to keep snack foods around the house that are healthy and easy to prepare. This will significantly reduce the amount of junk that they ingest and since this is the place where you can control what they do eat, then you should take full advantage of it.

In addition, you should encourage your teenager to eat breakfast every morning, no matter how small the amount, as this is the most important meal of the day and it will stop them from binging on junk food to satisfy their hunger during the day.

CHAPTER 4- GETTING RID OF THE PIMPLES

The pimples that teenage girls get when they enter puberty are usually a great source of embarrassment to them. Then spend a lot of time obsessing over them and trying to find ways and means in which to get rid of them as quickly as they can. The hormonal changes in their bodies are usually the culprit for these acnes on a girl's face as she goes through puberty.

This is so due to the fact that as their hormones fluctuate, so do the levels of their sebum, and this creates havoc by leading to the presence of acne all over their faces.

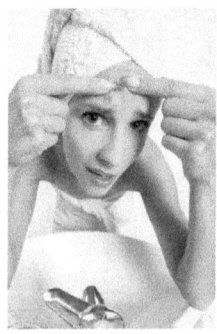

There are many types of acne treatments on the market; both over the counter and prescription types of acne treatment. Some teenage girls can treat their acne with over the counter acne treatments such as lotions, creams and benzoyl beroxide, and these you can find at your neighborhood drugstore or pharmacy.

Astringents are used by some teenagers to help with the excess oil in their skin. However, if they are over-used then it may dry out or irritate the skin.

Some teenagers have more serious acne issues that cannot be properly treated by over the counter drugs, and as such, they have to consult their doctor to get prescription medications to treat their ace problem. The oral medications they are usually prescribed should begin to take effect in a timely manner and stop the acne from becoming worse. Some doctors even prescribe contraceptives for some teenagers whose outbreaks are really bad, as that is the only way in which to control it.

Alternative health practitioners often recommend that teens and others who struggle with acne assess whether they're getting enough vitamins and minerals in their diet. Increasing their levels of vitamin A and/or zinc may help zits heal more quickly.

These holistic health care personnel usually recommend that teenagers who are having issues with acne find out if their minerals and vitamin levels are where it should be. If they are not, then they would suggest that they increase their intake of vitamin A as this will assist in treating their acne.

CHAPTER 5- GROWING BREASTS WHAT YOU SHOULD KNOW

Some teenage girls are very excited to start developing breast. However, there are some teenage girls who worry a lot about them; about how big they will grow and how they will look. The development of breasts is actually one of the very first signs of puberty in a girl. Breast growth can start as early as seven or eight years old, but there are others who do not start to do so until they turn thirteen or fourteen.

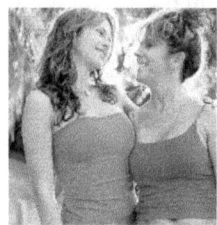

Their breasts will go through growth stages between the next five or six years until the teenager gets to be age seventeen or eighteen. Hereditary is usually a big determining factor as to how large a woman's breasts will eventually be.

Breasts are made up of ducts, fat, milk glands and connective tissue. The breast tissue of the teenage girl is usually dense and firm and gets more fatty and softer as they get older but the breasts have no muscle tissue. A woman's breasts are designed by nature to generate milk for their future children. However, in modern societies, the breasts are also seen as being sexually attractive and a big sign of a woman's femininity and sexuality.

When the breasts first begin to grow, it has a bud-like look, with small bumps appearing behind each of your nipples. The nipples will usually feel quite tender. As it gets bigger, the nipples and the areola will begin to get bigger and darker. After this, the rest of the breast will begin to grow. They will start out by looking pointy and then will become fuller and rounder as they get bigger.

14

Teenagers will usually start off by wearing what is called a training bra. These help to cover their pointy nipples and to give their growing breasts the support that they need. Sports bras are also recommended for girls who are just beginning to wear braziers. If the teenager's breasts are a little bigger than usual, then an underwire bra may be better for them as it would offer them much more support.

Some teenagers develop breasts very early and also have health issues with the size of their breasts. This is so when the breasts are too large that it sometimes cause a huge strain on their backs and cause their backs to curve and/or to cause them pain even when they wear the most supportive braziers that can be found on the market.

Sometimes they "grow into" their breast size, but there are other times when their breasts are just too big for their body structure and may call for breast reduction surgery in order to get their breasts down to a size that their body frame can comfortably carry around.

Some teenagers are very proud of their breasts; feeling grown up and excited about getting to wear a bra. However, there are those who are very subconscious about their breasts, especially if they are very large and draw way too much attention to them. Teenage boys can be very pesky and can torment teenage girls about their breasts and if the girl is already not comfortable with her breasts, then this will just make the situation much worse for her. Some girls have even been known to either wear baggy clothes to hide their bigger-sized breasts or to actually tie down their breasts so that they do not appear to be as big as they really are.

This can have a very negative impact on their self-esteem and can also cause health issues since they will be using whatever they are utilizing to tie down their breasts all the time while they are outside the comforts of their own home as this can lead to circulation issues as well as welts all over their chests, breasts and backs.

Sometimes surgery is necessary, while at other times they just need to visit a chiropractor who will help them to deal with the issues they are having with the pain in their back.

CHAPTER 6- YOUR REPRODUCTIVE SYSTEM : HOW IT WORKS FOR GIRLS

A woman's major reproductive tissues include her fallopian tubes, her ovaries as well as her womb and her vagina. As mentioned in the first chapter, the reproductive system is one of the aspects of a girl's entrance into puberty.

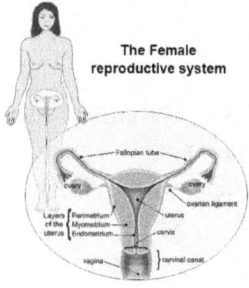

The hormones, which are chemicals that form in the body, are circulated in the blood and that are generated by the pituitary gland and the brain are usually in control of the functioning of these tissues. The production of breast milk, the menstrual cycle and pregnancy are controlled by these hormones. They are also responsible for the preparation of the walls of the uterus so that it can nourish and hold an egg that has been fertilized each month.

The sex hormones of the female also make a contribution to the general health of the liver, heart, and bones as well as a number of other tissues. During the period of pregnancy, there will be a production of the human chorionic gonadotropin (hCG) that helps the body to support a pregnancy until the woman has given birth.

What a lot of females do not know is that she is actually born with all the eggs she will have in her lifetime. As such, if these eggs are destroyed, they are not replaceable. When she gets to puberty, her menstrual cycles begin and the flow will usually last for only a few days.

Each new cycles brings with it the maturing of a new egg and after about two and three weeks the ovum; which is what the matured egg is called, is sent from the ovary and then carried by one of the fallopian tubes and if there is sexual activity during this time, then fertilization of the egg is possible.

However, if fertilization does not take place, then the egg will be broken up and will leave the body as the menstrual flow in that month after being in the fallopian tube for approximately two weeks.

CHAPTER 7- WHY YOUR PERIOD IS SO IMPORTANT FOR GIRLS

The menstrual cycle is an important part of the female reproductive system as alluded to in the previous chapter. In relation to a girl that is going through puberty, this is quite significant since it signifies her ability to now be able to become pregnant and to carry a child. A girl that is going through puberty can start her period from age eleven or twelve, but it is also normal for her to start her period anywhere between eight and sixteen years of age.

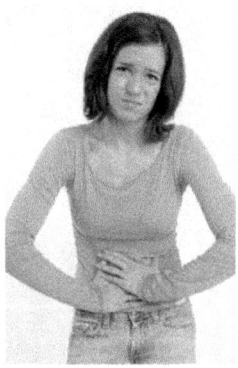

If a girl has not started to menstruate by the age of sixteen or about three years after she begins to grow breasts, then the parent, guardian or caregiver should take her to see a doctor so that they can figure out what is happening in her body.

Even though the symptoms associated with menstruating can be very difficult for some girls, having a menstrual cycle is actually an indication that the body is working in the way it should be working and that when she is ready, she should be able to have a child; barring any other kinds of factors that will prevent her from conceiving that may become apparent in the future.

The flow of your period can be light, medium or heavy and can be different in color; ranging from light to dark red. Most periods begin heavy and then eventually taper off at the end of the cycle. Your period usually last for between 3 and 5 days but can also have a menstrual cycle that is shorter or longer than 3 to 5 days. It is also normal if you do not have your period the same number of days every month during the first years of getting your period.

The menstrual cycle is what prepares the uterus for pregnancy and provides not just a place for the egg to live and grow for nine months, but also the nutrients that the egg will need to live to viability and then be delivered as a healthy baby after being fertilized by the sperm. The period also serves as a cleaning agent for the body. As such, a girl should avoid taking contraceptives to stop her cycle or to limit her cycles as this negatively affects the natural operation of the body.

CHAPTER 8- WHAT YOU NEED TO KNOW ABOUT BOYS

It is important for girls to know that they will be attracted to boys as this is the way that nature intends it to be. As such, they will have little crushes and even fall in love with them. It is also natural for them to have sexual feelings as again, this is how we are created. However, it is imperative for girls to know that when they enter puberty that they will be able to become pregnant if they have sexual intercourse with a boy, even if they are having sex for the very first time.

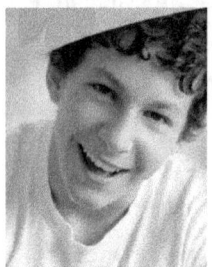

Girls also need to know that boys usually mature at a slower rate than girls and therefore may not be mentally and emotionally prepared to take on certain responsibilities. With that in mind, girls should try to stay away from getting involved sexually with a boy, as the only thing that will protect you one hundred percent from becoming pregnant is abstinence.

In addition, the fact is that a boy can be very interested in you this minute and then act as if you do not even exist the next; passing you in the hall ways at school and not even saying hi.

In addition to the foregoing, girls also need to know that boys are just as shy and unsure of themselves during puberty as they are, and that a lot of what they do is simply bravado that they use in order to hide their own fears and insecurities. They will sometimes spread rumors about having sex with a girl so that they can gain popularity and feel important among their peers.

Additionally, some boys will tease a girl un-mercilessly when he likes her a lot but do not know how else to express it, or is afraid of being rejected by her. It is important for girls to know that teen age are just human beings with their own insecurities and are just learning about the world the same way that they are.

CHAPTER 9- WHAT EVERY TEENAGE GIRL SHOULD KNOW ABOUT SEX

Psychologists will tell you that teenage girls are just not mentally or emotionally equipped to engage in sexual intercourse. The act of sex can be a very overwhelming even for adults much less for teenagers.

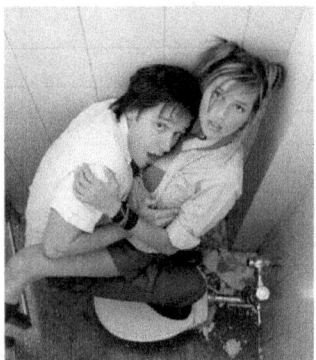

There is always a lot to be concerned about, to know and to work on so that nothing will go wrong such as pregnancy and/or sexually transmitted diseases. Whether or not a teenage girl is sexually active, it is imperative for them to know the facts about sex and all the implications that do come with it.

Every teenage girl should be made aware of the fact that sex involves their bodies as well as their emotions. As such, they will not be able to just have sex with a boy or boys and not be hurt emotionally when they do not talk to them in school the next day or they tell their friends and they are being called all kinds of terrible names all around their school; damaging their reputation.

In addition, when you have sex with a boy it will not make them love you or become committed to you just because you have given him your body. Sex comes with a whole lot of responsibilities that teenagers are not ready to take on at this early stage of their life. It should not be used as a bargaining tool, as a way to spite another boy, to rebel against your parents or to prove how grown up you are.

If you are a teenage girl that is already engaging in sexual intercourse, you should know that there are actually laws having to do with you being at the age of consent for engaging in the sex act and even about the type of sex you can have. This means that sex is a very serious undertaking and not something to be taken too lightly.

Many persons are against giving teenagers contraceptives in the form of condoms or taking them to get put on birth control by their doctors. However, the fact is that many teenagers are indulging in sexual intercourse and have gotten pregnant and gotten very dangerous sexually transmitted diseases that have changed their lives in a negative way forever, due to the fact that they have indulged in un-protected sex.

In addition, it is also imperative for her to know that even if she is using contraceptives that do not mean that she is completely safe from becoming pregnant or contracting a sexually transmitted disease as condoms do break and other birth control methods also do fail sometimes. If she is on the pill and misses even one pill, she can still end up getting pregnant this way.

The teenage girl should also be told that oral sex is sex too and that there are actually sexually transmitted diseases that you can get while engaging in this type of sex. These sexually transmitted diseases can be permanent such as HIV and AIDS.

The first time a girl has sex is usually very painful as the erect penis will have to break her hymen before her vagina can be penetrated and she will bleed during and sometimes after the se act. The hymen is a membrane that partly covers or that surrounds the vaginal opening and is a part of the external genitalia.

ABOUT THE AUTHOR

Dana Tebow has worked with teenage and pre-puberty girls for as long as she can remember. She sees this as such a very important time in a girl's life and has always thought that it was crucial that they be given the proper tools and the requisite information so that they can enter this scary and sometimes confusing time not being scared due to the unknown or not being prepared for what their body as well as their emotions will go through.

She knows too well what not having the necessary information can cause to the life of a teenager as the lack of information is what caused her to be a mother of twins when she was only sixteen years old as she thought that she could not get pregnant the first time she had sex, which is exactly what happened to her.

She loves her children, but she was not prepared to raise children when she was just a child herself, and it took away her childhood and her opportunity to just be a child. It also set back her plans for college and her career for more than a decade. However, she has no regrets as she has gotten to do all the things that she ever wanted to do, like going to college and getting a degree.

However, her experience as a teenage mother greatly impacted on her career choice, since she wanted to be an attorney, or thought she did as a teenager, but she ended up becoming a social worker, as she wanted to be able to talk to girls about entering puberty and all it will mean to their lives..